Sweat and Success

A Journey to Fitness

By: **Andrew G. Finch.**

Copyright © 2023 by Andrew G. Finch

Terms of Use:

By accessing or using this book, you agree to the following terms and conditions:

1. This book is provided for informational and educational purposes only. The author is not a licensed medical or fitness professional, and the content is not intended as a substitute for professional advice, diagnosis, or treatment.
2. The author and publisher make no representations or warranties about the accuracy, completeness, or suitability of the information contained in this book. Use the information at your own risk.
3. Any reliance you place on the information in this book is strictly at your own discretion. You should consult with a qualified healthcare provider or fitness professional before starting any fitness program or making significant changes to your lifestyle.

4. The author and publisher shall not be liable for any direct, indirect, incidental, consequential, or special damages arising out of or in any way connected with the use or misuse of this book or the information contained herein.
5. This book may contain links to third-party websites or resources for additional information. The author and publisher are not responsible for the content, availability, or accuracy of such external sites or resources.
6. All trademarks, registered trademarks, and service marks mentioned in this book are the property of their respective owners.
7. Unauthorized distribution, reproduction, or sharing of this book, in whole or in part, is strictly prohibited and may result in legal action.

Disclaimer:

The information presented in this book is based on the author's personal knowledge and research as of the date of publication. While every effort has been made to provide accurate and up-to-date information, the author and publisher make no representations or warranties regarding the completeness, accuracy, or applicability of the information for any specific purpose.

This book is not intended to provide medical, fitness, or nutritional advice. The author is not a licensed medical or fitness professional, and the content is for informational purposes only. You should consult with a qualified healthcare provider or fitness professional before starting any fitness program, making dietary changes, or following any recommendations in this book.

The author and publisher shall not be held responsible for any loss, injury, or damage allegedly arising from any information or recommendations provided in this book. Use the information at your own discretion and risk.

Any testimonials or success stories presented in this book are individual experiences and do not guarantee similar results for all readers. Your results may vary based on your individual circumstances, dedication, and adherence to fitness and nutrition guidelines.

By using this book, you acknowledge that you have read, understood, and agreed to the terms and disclaimers outlined herein.

Table of Contents

Sweat and Success

Introduction:

Our health frequently takes a backseat in today's fast-paced society, where our schedules are frequently driven by never-ending to-do lists and constant stress. But what if I told you that starting a fitness adventure could be the key to changing both your life and your physical appearance? Welcome to "Sweat and Success: A Journey to Fitness," a thorough manual that will lead you on a transformational journey to a healthier, happier version of yourself.

This book explores the remarkable synergy between the mind and body, not merely how to build a lean physique. It's about overcoming self-doubt, escaping the restrictions of a sedentary existence, and embracing a refreshing change.

Over the course of the next 15 chapters, we'll go deeply into the realm of fitness, covering topics like setting reasonable goals, dispelling popular beliefs, creating effective workout routines, and cultivating a mindset that supports success. We'll cater to the requirements of people of all ages and fitness levels to make sure that everyone can participate in this voyage.

Turn the page now and let's start on this amazing adventure to a healthier, more energetic life if you're prepared to work up a sweat, conquer challenges, and reveal the best version of yourself.

Chapter 1

The Path to a Healthier You

Starting in the first chapter of "Sweat and Success: A Journey to Fitness," we travel along the road to a healthier you. You will be guided through the first steps in this chapter, assisting you in setting the groundwork for your fitness journey.

The choice to alter.

Making the decision to change is the first and most important step on the road to fitness. It all starts with one crucial choice, whether your goal is to lose extra weight, gain muscle, or simply enhance your general well-being.

Choosing Your Fitness Objectives

Once you've made the decision to change, it's time to make specific, doable fitness objectives. Your roadmap will be these objectives, which will help you stay motivated and on task while you travel. To make sure your goals are clear and attainable, we'll dive in-depth with the SMART (Specific, Measurable, Achievable, Relevant, Time-bound) goal-setting framework.

How to Evaluate Your Fitness Level Currently

You must first comprehend where you are right now to grasp where you're going. We'll look at several techniques, such as body measurements, strength testing, and cardiovascular evaluations, to determine your present level of fitness. You may adjust your workout routine to meet your specific needs with the use of this knowledge.

Choosing a motivation

Any fitness journey that is effective is fueled by motivation. We'll study strategies to keep a high level of motivation throughout your fitness transition as well as the main sources of motivation, ranging from enhancing health to boosting confidence.

Building a Support Network

Having a strong support system around you can have a big impact on your success. We'll talk about how having support from friends, family, or exercise partners who can hold you accountable for your health goals is crucial.

starting the process

It's now time to take that crucial first step after making the decision to change, setting goals, determining your fitness level, igniting your motivation, and putting your support system in place. We'll offer advice on picking the best exercise program and making a routine that works with your lifestyle.

Be mindful of the fact that change requires time, commitment, and work as you set out on this road. The first chapter of "Sweat and Success: A Journey to Fitness" is where the road to a healthy you begin. Embrace it with tenacity and the awareness that there will be transformation and success on the way.

Chapter 2

Creating SMART Fitness Objectives

You bravely decided in Chapter 1 to transform your life via exercise. In "Sweat and Success: A Journey to Fitness," Chapter 2, we'll go into more detail about the skill of goal planning. Setting realistic fitness goals is essential because they act as your compass and direct you in the right direction.

Setting SMART Objectives

SMART goals are time-bound, relevant, specified, measurable, and achievable. Let's analyze each component in turn:

➢ Specific: Your aim should be distinct and well-defined. Don't just state, "I want to lose weight," but be specific about how much and when you want to lose it.

➢ Measurable: Your objective should have metrics that can be measured. If your objective is to increase strength, for example, you should be able to track it by keeping track of the weights you lift or the number of repetitions you can complete.

➢ Realistic and doable: Your objective should be attainable. Setting impossible standards may result in frustration. Setting goals that stretch you yet are attainable is crucial.

➢ Relevant: Your purpose should be pertinent to your overall fitness ambitions and ideals. It needs to be significant to you personally and benefit your long-term wellbeing.

➢ Time-bound: Your objective ought to have a due date. Having a deadline aid in maintaining commitment and attention.

various fitness objectives

Fitness objectives can be divided into several categories, including:

- **Weight Loss Objectives:** If your main goal is to lose weight, establish a reasonable benchmark based on your present weight and body composition.
- **Strength goals** are focused on enhancing your physical power, whether you desire to bench press a specific weight or complete a specific number of pull-ups.
- **Goals for enhancing** your stamina and cardiovascular fitness are considered endurance goals. Examples

include cycling a particular route or running a specified distance.

- **Goals for Flexibility:** Improving your mobility and flexibility is essential for avoiding injuries and maintaining general health.
- **Goals for your diet:** such as increasing the number of servings of fruits and vegetables you consume each day or cutting back on sugar, are known as nutrition goals.

Short-term versus long-term goals

A combination of long-term and short-term goals will help you on your fitness path. Long-term objectives, like finishing a marathon or dropping a large amount of weight, give direction. Short-term objectives let you take achievable steps toward your long-term vision, such as setting weekly exercise goals or making nutritional adjustments.

Monitoring Progress

Tracking your development is crucial for success in your fitness quest. We'll look at a variety of tools, such fitness apps, journals, and body measures, for tracking your progress. Observing your progress can be quite inspiring.

Changing Goals

To achieve your fitness goals, flexibility is essential. Your priorities and circumstances may change since life is erratic. We'll go over how to modify your objectives as necessary without straying from your long-term fitness objectives.

As you begin Chapter 2, keep in mind that the foundation of your journey is creating sensible fitness goals. These goals will help you stay on track, inspired, and enthusiastic about the changes that are coming. So, let's keep pursuing your goal of "sweat and success."

Chapter 3

Getting to Know Your Nutrition: Fueling Your Body

In Chapter 3 of "Sweat and Success: A Journey to Fitness," we'll talk about nutrition, which is an important aspect of your fitness journey. Your body is a precisely honed machine, and the fuel you give it may have a huge impact on how well you perform and how successful you are.

Nutrition: Its Importance

Giving your body the necessary nutrients, it needs to function at its best is what nutrition is all about. It's not just about what you eat. Understanding nutrition is essential whether your objective is to reduce weight, build muscle, or simply maintain a healthy lifestyle.

dietary macro- and micronutrients

The two primary groups of nutrients are macronutrients and micronutrients.

1. Carbohydrates, proteins, and lipids are macronutrients. Each has a special function in your diet. Energy is provided by carbohydrates, muscle

repair and growth is aided by proteins, and various biological processes require fats.

2. Micronutrients are vitamins and minerals required for good health in general. These include minerals like calcium, iron, and zinc as well as vitamins like A, C, and D.

A healthy diet

A balanced diet offers all the essential elements in the appropriate amounts. We'll talk about how eating a variety of foods will help you acquire a variety of nutrients in your diet.

When to eat

You're eating habits, including when and how much, can affect your fitness objectives. We'll explore ideas including meal frequency, nutrition before and after exercise, and intermittent fasting.

Hydration

Your overall health and sports performance depend on you being hydrated appropriately. We'll talk about the value of drinking water and how to stay well hydrated all day.

Meal preparation

A crucial technique for preserving a balanced diet is meal planning. We'll give you advice and resources to assist you in organizing and preparing wholesome meals that support your fitness objectives.

Unique Diets

We'll examine how to modify several special diets, such as vegetarian, vegan, ketogenic, and paleo diets, for those who have dietary restrictions or specific fitness goals.

Avoiding Typical Nutrition Errors

There are many myths about nutrition, which makes it difficult to understand. We'll bust common misconceptions and hazards so you can make wise decisions.

seeking advice from a professional

A trained dietitian or nutritionist can be quite helpful if you're unaware of your nutritional requirements or have special health issues.

You'll have a firm understanding of how nutrition is crucial to your fitness journey by the end of Chapter 3. With this information at your disposal, you'll be better able to make educated food decisions that support your objectives and open the door to a healthier, fitter you. Let's continue your studies in the fields of diet and fitness with "Sweat and Success."

Chapter 4

Strengthening Your Foundation Through Strength Training

Thank you for reading Chapter 4 of "Sweat and Success: A Journey to Fitness." We'll delve into the fascinating world of strength training in this chapter. Building a strong foundation of strength involves more than just becoming physically stronger; it also involves enhancing your general health and well-being.

Why Strength Training Is Beneficial

Beyond only increasing muscular mass, strength training has a wide range of advantages:

- Increasing muscle mass can increase metabolism since muscle burns more calories at rest than fat does.
- Enhanced functional strength makes it easier for you to carry out regular duties and lowers your chance of injury.
- Strengthening Your Bones: Resistance training can strengthen your bones and lower your chances of osteoporosis.

- ➢ Strength training has been demonstrated to lessen the signs of anxiety and sadness.
- ➢ Strength training can improve your athletic performance, whether you're a professional athlete or just play sports for fun.

Starting a Strength Training Program

- **Prior to lifting weights:** it's critical to comprehend the following basic ideas:
- **Exercise Technique:** Developing good exercise technique is essential to avoiding injuries.
- **Resistance:** We'll look at many forms of resistance, including bodyweight exercises, machines, resistance bands, and free weights.
- **Training Splits:** We'll talk about different training splits, including full-body exercises, splits for the upper and lower bodies, and programs tailored to particular muscle groups.

Creating a Workout Schedule

A few essential components go into designing a strength training program that is well-rounded:

- ➢ Exercise selection is the process of selecting the best workouts to grow the muscle groups you desire.

- ➢ Progressive Overload: Constantly pushing your muscles to their limits by gradually increasing the weight or intensity of your workouts.
- ➢ Recovery: Time for muscular growth and recovery is essential for improvement.

Strength Training for Various Objectives

Your strength training program may change based on your fitness objectives. We'll discuss:

- muscular Building: We'll talk about hypertrophy training for people wishing to increase their muscular mass.
- Gains in Strength: If you want to get stronger, we'll discuss regimens that are tailored to that goal.
- Exercises that are centered on endurance are the best for increasing muscle stamina.

Preventing Common Errors

We'll also point out typical errors newcomers make when strength training and explain how to avoid them.

Progress Monitoring

Monitoring your gains in strength is both inspiring and crucial for maximizing your training program. We'll cover techniques for keeping tabs on your lifts and establishing objectives.

Considerations for Safety

Strength training places a high priority on safety. We'll offer advice on how to avoid injuries and what to do if you experience pain or discomfort while working out.

You'll have a firm grasp of the fundamentals of strength training and how to apply it to your fitness journey by the end of Chapter 4. Whether you're a beginner or have some lifting expertise, this chapter will provide you with the tools you need to create a solid foundation and open the door to a fitter, healthier self in "Sweat and Success."

Chapter 5

Getting Your Heart Pumping with Cardiovascular Fitness

Thank you for reading Chapter 5 of "Sweat and Success: A Journey to Fitness." We'll look at the crucial elements of cardiovascular fitness in this chapter. Cardio exercises are essential for increasing your endurance and overall health in addition to getting your heart rate up.

Getting to Know Cardiovascular Fitness

Exercises that raise your heart rate and breathing for a prolonged length of time are the emphasis of cardiovascular fitness, also known as cardio or aerobic exercise. Numerous advantages of these exercises include:

> ➤ Improved Heart Health: Cardiovascular exercises build up and improve the function of your heart muscle.
> ➤ Improved Lung Function: This increases your ability to take in more oxygen.
> ➤ Exercises that burn calories, such as cardio, can help people lose or maintain their weight.
> ➤ Cardiovascular exercise releases endorphins, which lower stress and lift mood.

Cardiovascular Exercise Types

There are many different cardio exercises you may do, so pick ones you prefer. Typical types include:

- **Running** is an efficient technique to raise your heart rate, whether you favor jogging or sprinting.
- **Cycling:** Either indoors or outside, cycling is a low-impact activity that is easy on the joints.
- **Swimming:** Swimming is easy on the joints and offers a full-body workout.
- **Dancing:** Dancing is a great way to increase your heart rate while enhancing balance and coordination.
- **Jumping rope** is a straightforward but efficient aerobic exercise that can be performed virtually anyplace.

Cardiovascular targets

Setting goals for your cardiovascular workouts is crucial, just like it is for strength training. We'll go over how to set objectives for your cardiovascular health, your speed, or both.

Developing cardio exercises

It takes careful consideration to choose the proper intensity, duration, and frequency while creating a cardio workout. We'll look at how to design cardio workouts that suit your objectives and degree of fitness.

High-intensity interval training, or HIIT

A popular and effective cardio technique known as HIIT comprises short bursts of intense exercise followed by quick rest periods. We'll go through the advantages of HIIT and how to work it into your daily schedule.

Cardio Long-Distance

We'll offer training advice and winning tactics for people interested in long-distance running, cycling, or other endurance sports.

Safety Measures

Cardio activities require a high level of safety, especially if you're pushing yourself to the edge. We'll talk about how to avoid injuries and what to do if you feel uncomfortable while going out.

Cross-Training

To avoid boredom and lower your risk of overuse problems, cross-training entails combining a variety of aerobic exercises into your daily regimen. We'll go over cross-training correctly.

You'll have a thorough understanding of cardiovascular fitness and how to apply it to your fitness journey by the end of Chapter 5. This chapter of "Sweat and Success" will lead you to success whether your goal is to enhance your heart health, increase endurance, or simply take advantage of the mental and physical advantages of cardiac exercise.

Chapter 6

Mobility and Flexibility are Essential for Injury Prevention

Thank you for reading Chapter 6 of "Sweat and Success: A Journey to Fitness." We'll examine the sometimes disregarded yet crucial facets of flexibility and mobility in this chapter. These components are crucial for improving your daily comfort and performance in addition to helping you avoid injuries.

Recognizing Mobility and Flexibility

- **Your muscles' flexibility** is their capacity to stretch and extend. It is crucial for preserving your joints' complete range of motion.
- **Mobility:** Pays attention to the range of mobility in your joints. It concerns the condition and flexibility of the joint capsule, tendons, and ligaments.

Benefits of Flexibility and Mobility Injury Prevention:

- ➤ By keeping your joints flexible and mobile, you lower your risk of sprains, strains, and other injuries from happening during exercises or regular activities.

- ➢ Better Posture: Greater flexibility and mobility help people maintain better posture, which lowers their chance of developing chronic pain and discomfort.
- ➢ enhanced Performance: Increased mobility can result in enhanced performance and technique in sports and fitness activities.
- ➢ Pain relief: Flexibility exercises can lessen the likelihood of muscle imbalances that cause pain and soothe aching muscles.

Exercises for mobility vs. flexibility

We'll discuss how to combine mobility and flexibility exercises into your regimen as well as the differences between the two.

Practicing stretches

Stretching is a key step in increasing flexibility. We'll look at different stretching methods, such as proprioceptive neuromuscular facilitation (PNF) stretching and dynamic and static stretching.

Rolling in the foam and self-myofascial release

Self-myofascial release and foam rolling are techniques for releasing muscular tension and knots, which enhance flexibility and mobility.

Pilates and yoga

Yoga and Pilates both place a strong emphasis on core stability, suppleness, and flexibility. We'll talk about how these habits can help you achieve your fitness goals.

Flexibility and Mobility in Your Daily Routine

We'll offer advice on how to include mobility and flexibility drills in both stand-alone workouts and your warm-up and cool-down routines.

evaluating and monitoring development

It's crucial to evaluate and monitor your flexibility and mobility development, just like with other fitness-related areas, to detect changes over time.

Considerations for Safety

When working on flexibility and movement, safety comes first. To avoid injuries, we'll talk about typical mistakes and how to avoid them.

You'll understand the importance of flexibility and mobility in your fitness journey by the end of Chapter 6. You'll have a toolkit of workouts and methods at your disposal to increase your range of motion, lower your chance of injury, and enhance your general physical health. Let's thus carry on your efforts to become a healthier, more adaptable, and mobile self in "Sweat and Success."

Chapter 7

Fitness Psychology: Maintaining Motivation

Thank you for reading Chapter 7 of "Sweat and Success: A Journey to Fitness." We'll examine the critical part psychology plays in your journey toward fitness in this chapter. The keys to reaching your fitness objectives include continuing to be motivated, conquering challenges, and keeping a good outlook.

The Mind-Body Relationship

Your physical performance and outcomes are significantly influenced by your thinking. Long-term success requires an understanding of the psychology of fitness.

Motivation

We'll explore the science of motivation and the inherent and extrinsic motivations for working toward your fitness objectives. Knowing what motivates you can help you maintain your commitment when times are difficult.

Visualizing Your Goals

Utilizing visualization techniques can help you achieve your fitness objectives. We'll lead you through exercises that will help you clearly picture your accomplishments and strengthen your dedication to your goals.

Positivity in Oneself

It matters how you speak to yourself. We'll talk about the value of developing a constructive internal dialogue and offer techniques to deal with unfavorable self-talk.

Overcoming Obstacles and Plateaus

Any fitness quest will inevitably encounter barriers and plateaus. We'll look at typical obstacles, including getting bored with your workouts and hitting weight loss plateaus, and talk about how to get beyond them.

decrease of stress and mindfulness

Your fitness development may be halted by stress. To keep you calm and concentrated, we'll cover stress-reduction techniques and mindfulness.

The impact of routines

Sticking to your regimen can be made much easier by developing healthy fitness habits. We'll talk about how habits are formed and offer advice for forming healthy workout habits.

Responsibility and assistance

Your motivation can be significantly impacted by your support network. We'll look at ways that your friends, family, or exercise partners can help you stay on track.

Monitoring Development and Honoring Success

Staying motivated requires regularly monitoring your progress and acknowledging your accomplishments, no matter how minor. We'll talk about keeping a log of your progress and rewarding yourself for your efforts.

Managing setbacks

Failures occur along the way. We'll offer techniques for overcoming failures and avoiding discouragement.

consulting a professional

Don't be afraid to seek out expert advice from a therapist or counselor if you discover that your fitness journey is causing you to struggle with motivation or to have mental health issues.

You'll have a thorough understanding of the psychological aspects of fitness and how to use your mind's power to stay motivated and get through obstacles by the end of Chapter 7. self will be prepared to continue your path to a fitter, healthier self in "Sweat and Success" if you have the appropriate attitude.

Chapter 8

Overcoming Obstacles and Plateaus

In Chapter 8 of "Sweat and Success: A Journey to Fitness," we'll go more deeply into the inevitable plateaus and difficulties you'll face while working toward health. Although these times might be frustrating, they also present chances for development and change.

Recognizing Plateaus

There are times when you seem to be making no progress at all despite continuing to work hard. They can happen in a variety of fitness-related areas, such as weight loss, strength development, or endurance enhancement.

the typical causes of plateaus

We'll look at some of the typical causes of plateaus, like:

- ➢ Your body will adjust to your exercise regimen with time, decreasing its effectiveness.
- ➢ Dietary factors, such as ingesting too many or too few calories, might contribute to plateaus.
- ➢ Overtraining: Platting can result from pushing your body too far without getting enough rest.

Techniques for Breaking Plateaus

It takes a combination of persistence, adaptation, and deliberate changes to break past plateaus. We'll go over practical tactics like:

> ➤ Progressive overload: challenging your body by gradually raising the intensity or complexity of your workouts.
>
> ➤ Altering the workout's frequency, duration, or workouts will keep your body on its toes.
>
> ➤ Nutritional Modifications: Tailoring your diet to meet your objectives, whether it means changing your calorie intake or the time of your nutrients,
>
> ➤ Making sure you have enough rest and recovery time will help your body heal and develop.
>
> ➤ Mental fortitude: Remaining upbeat and persistent when motivation stalls

Continued Consistency

For plateaus to be broken, consistency is essential. We'll offer techniques for keeping your dedication and consistency even in the face of difficulties.

Considering the Long-Term Journey

A natural aspect of any fitness program are plateaus. You can stay motivated by remembering that they're only transitory and a component of your overall development.

Having reasonable expectations

We'll stress how crucial it is to have realistic expectations about your fitness goals and the amount of time it will take to reach them.

tracking and recognizing modest victories

Small triumphs along the way can serve as inspiration to push past plateaus, so it's important to acknowledge and celebrate them.

Looking for Advice

It may occasionally be necessary to hire a personal trainer or other fitness specialist to help you break a plateau. Don't be afraid to ask for help when you need it.

By the end of Chapter 8, you'll have the skills and tactics necessary to get past obstacles in your fitness path, such as plateaus. Remember that plateaus are not obstacles; rather, they are chances for you to grow, change, and eventually reach new heights on your journey to a healthier, more fit version of yourself in "Sweat and Success."

Chapter 9

Monitoring Your Success: Monitoring Your Progress

The topic of measuring and recording your progress is covered in detail in Chapter 9 of "Sweat and Success: A Journey to Fitness." You'll remain inspired and committed to your goals if you can see concrete proof of your successes.

The Value of Monitoring Progress

A map of your fitness journey can be had by tracking your progress. It facilitates:

- Keep your motivation up: Observing progress can increase your self-assurance and drive.
- Make educated choices: Data can help you modify your diet and exercise routine.
- Celebrate Your Success: Small victories add up to big successes.
- Finding Plateaus: You'll be able to tell when your progress stalls or slows down.

Various Methods for Monitoring Progress

We'll look at several ways to monitor your fitness progress:

- ➤ Tracking changes in your weight, body fat percentage, and physical characteristics
- ➤ Fitness Tracking Apps: Using wearables or fitness tracking apps to measure workouts, steps, and other information.
- ➤ Measuring your exercise performance by keeping track of the weights you lift, the distances you run, or the number of repetitions you can complete,
- ➤ Before-and-after pictures: Seeing tangible proof of your progress can be inspiring.
- ➤ Fitness journals: Recording your workouts, diet, and emotions in detail.
- ➤ Test your level of fitness on occasion by putting yourself through a series of exercises or challenges.

setting objectives and standards

We'll talk about how important it is to develop clear, attainable goals and benchmarks. Benchmarks are midway points that show you are moving in the right direction toward your overall fitness goals.

Tracking Progress Frequently

Depending on your goals, you can choose how frequently you monitor your progress. We'll offer instructions on when and how to accurately gauge your development.

Using Regression to Encourage You

Even though they are frustrating, plateaus can serve as inspiration. We'll demonstrate how to evaluate plateaus and draw conclusions from them.

Keeping Your Focus

It's critical to approach measuring your progress objectively and to not let tiny setbacks demoralize you. We'll offer advice on how to keep a fair viewpoint.

obtaining professional evaluation

At times, getting a professional evaluation from a health care physician, nutritionist, or fitness trainer can provide insightful information about your current and potential development areas.

You'll have a thorough understanding of how to efficiently track your fitness improvement by the end of Chapter 9. With these methods and tactics at your disposal, you'll be better able to maintain motivation, make wise choices, and recognize your accomplishments as you work toward becoming a healthier, more fit version of yourself in "Sweat and Success."

Chapter 10

Healthy Routines for Life

Chapter 10 of "Sweat and Success: A Journey to Fitness" discusses the significance of forming lifelong healthy habits. To attain your fitness goals, you must adopt a sustained, healthy lifestyle in addition to a certain weight or level of strength.

The impact of routines

The foundation of our daily existence is comprised of habits. You can experience long-lasting, beneficial changes in your fitness level and general well-being by forming healthy habits.

Creation of Habits

We'll talk about how to develop and maintain healthy habits as well as the science behind habit formation.

habits in nutrition

Maintaining a healthy diet is essential for long-term success. We'll look at methods for:

> ➤ Paying attention to your food and eating habits is known as mindful eating.

- ➤ Creating balanced meals and snacks according to a food plan
- ➤ Portion Control: Limit your intake by controlling your portion sizes.
- ➤ Make sure you drink enough water throughout the day to stay hydrated.

Exercise Routines

Exercise regularly is a crucial habit for keeping fit. We'll talk about how to:

- ➤ Create an exercise regimen that works with your lifestyle by establishing a routine.
- ➤ Find things You Truly Enjoy: To make exercise enjoyable rather than a chore, find things you truly enjoy.
- ➤ Stay Active: Include movement in your everyday routine by walking or climbing the stairs, for example.

Sleep Patterns

Sleeping well is crucial for recovery and general health. We'll look at methods for enhancing your sleeping patterns.

Stress Reduction

Your wellbeing depends on being able to manage your stress. To assist you effectively manage stress, we'll talk about time management, deep breathing, and meditation.

Making Informed Decisions

Making deliberate, healthy decisions in all facets of your life, such as eating and exercising, can be facilitated by mindfulness practice.

Getting Over Obstacles

Setbacks are a part of the journey toward developing good habits. We'll offer tips for picking up the pieces following mistakes.

Social Assistance

Your healthy habits might be strengthened if you have a network of friends and family that support you. We'll talk about how to get family members involved in your fitness goals.

Keeping the Motivation

The key to long-term success is maintaining motivation. We'll talk about how developing healthy habits may motivate you.

Making a Customized Plan

We'll help you develop a unique strategy for forming and keeping sane habits that suit your lifestyle and fitness objectives.

You'll comprehend the value of healthy habits in your trip toward fitness by the end of Chapter 10 and how to develop them for a lifetime of wellbeing. These behaviors will not only assist you in achieving your present objectives but will also enable you to maintain your success and advance in "Sweat and Success."

Chapter 11

From teenagers to seniors, fitness is for everyone

In Chapter 11 of "Sweat and Success: A Journey to Fitness," we discuss the significance of fitness for people of all ages. Fitness is a lifelong journey that can bring health, vitality, and joy at every stage of life; it is not restricted to a certain age.

Youth Exercise

A healthy life can be built on a strong foundation of early fitness. We'll talk about:

- Promoting sports and active play for children's physical development through physical activity
- Teen Fitness: Getting regular exercise while juggling schoolwork and extracurriculars.

Adult Exercise

Growing up presents its own set of difficulties and obligations. We'll look at:

- How to Maintain Fitness While Managing a Career and Family: Balancing Work and Fitness

> ➤ How to fit exercise into a hectic parenting schedule for parents who are fit.

Middle-aged fitness

Our fitness requirements may alter as we age. We'll talk about:

> ➤ Age-Related Weight Management: Techniques for Retaining a Healthy Weight
> ➤ Exercises to prevent muscle wasting and preserve bone density for strength and bone health.

Senior Exercise

For older people to retain their independence and quality of life, fitness is crucial. We'll look at:

> ➤ Exercises to prevent falls and injuries while maintaining balance.
> ➤ Techniques to Maintain Mobility and Decrease Joint Stiffness: Flexibility and Joint Health
> ➤ Seniors' cognitive performance and physical activity are related in terms of mental health.

Changing Exercises for Age

We'll offer advice on how to modify workouts for various age groups while considering specific requirements and limits.

Lifelong Fitness Benefits

Staying active throughout your life has several advantages, including bettering your physical and mental health and lengthening your life.

Maintaining Family Activity

A culture of health and wellbeing can be fostered by participating in fitness activities as a family for many generations.

Dispelling age-related rumors

We'll dispel popular misconceptions about fitness and aging, such the idea that you can't increase your strength or endurance as you age.

seeking advice from a professional

Working with a fitness expert or healthcare provider is crucial for safe and efficient exercise for people with special health concerns or age-related challenges.

You'll see by the end of Chapter 11 that fitness has no age restrictions. Fitness is a lifetime journey that may benefit everyone, whether you're a teenager aiming to establish a solid foundation, an adult juggling a hectic life, or a senior seeking to preserve vitality. Accept your individual fitness requirements and enjoy the journey to health and happiness in "Sweat and Success."

Chapter 12

Fitness Outside of the Gym: Alternative Sports and Outdoor Activities

Chapter 12 of "Sweat and Success: A Journey to Fitness" delves into the thrilling realm of outdoor adventures and non-traditional fitness pursuits. There are various ways to keep active and healthy while enjoying the great outdoors and participating in non-traditional workouts, even if the gym offers a solid foundation for fitness.

The Natural World

Fitness and adventure options abound in nature. We'll talk about a variety of outdoor activities, like:

- ➤ Hiking enhances cardiovascular health and leg strength while allowing you to explore trails and mountains.
- ➤ Cycling: Pedaling through beautiful scenery while getting some fitness
- ➤ Swimming is a great way to exercise your entire body while having fun in the water.
- ➤ Scaling cliffs and boulders to test your strength, agility, and problem-solving abilities is rock climbing.

> ➤ Paddling through rivers and lakes in a kayak or canoe builds core and upper body strength.

Mind/Body Techniques

The mind-body link is frequently emphasized in alternative exercise practices. We'll look at techniques like:

> ➤ Yoga: Using various yoga forms, you can improve your flexibility, balance, and mental clarity.
> ➤ Tai Chi: This flowing martial technique can help with balance, coordination, and relaxation.
> ➤ Pilates: boosting body awareness, strengthening the core, and enhancing posture.

Movement and dancing

Exercises including movement and dance are not only enjoyable, but also a great way to keep in shape. We'll talk about:

> ➤ Zumba: a high-intensity workout combining dance and aerobics.
> ➤ Ballet methods can be used in fitness for better posture and muscle tone.
> ➤ Using urban settings for agility and strength training is called parkour.

Exercise Challenges

Participating in obstacle courses and fitness challenges makes your training more exciting. We'll look at things like:

> ➤ Running through mud is a fun cardio and strength exercise known as "mud runs."
> ➤ Spartan races combine strenuous obstacles like rope climbs and spear throws with running.

Fitness that is inclusive and adapted

Regardless of one's physical capabilities, everyone can benefit from fitness. We'll talk about adaptive fitness exercises and programs that can meet different demands.

choosing a passion

Discovering activities, you actually enjoy is the secret to continuing to be active and dedicated to health. We'll offer advice on how to identify your fitness interests.

Considerations for Safety

When participating in outdoor adventures and alternative activities, safety must come first. We'll go over how to be ready, stay secure, and fully appreciate your exercise.

You'll have a fresh respect for the varied fitness industry outside of the gym by the end of Chapter 12. There are several ways to keep active and healthy while having fun, whether you love the outdoors, dancing, or are just trying to mix up your routine. In "Sweat and Success," embrace the adventure and unconventional activities that will help you succeed in your fitness goals.

Chapter 13

The Science of Recovery: Rejuvenating Your Body and Restoring It

Thank you for reading Chapter 13 of "Sweat and Success: A Journey to Fitness." This chapter will examine a crucial yet underappreciated component of recovery. Achieving your fitness objectives, avoiding injuries, and preserving your long-term well-being all depend on proper recovery.

Recognizing the significance of recovery

Recovery is the process through which your body recovers from and acclimates to the strain that exercise places on it. It includes the following aspects:

➤ Muscle Repair: Following a workout, recovery enables your muscles to recover and get stronger.
➤ Restoring energy: It tops out the reserves depleted during exercise.
➤ Injury Prevention: Ample healing lowers the incidence of acute injuries and helps prevent overuse injuries.
➤ Mental Rejuvenation: For mental health and motivation, recovery is also necessary.

types of healing

We'll talk about several types of recuperation, like:

> ➤ Active recovery: low-stress, low-intensity exercises like light yoga or strolling that increase blood flow.
> ➤ Complete rest, allowing your body to repair and replenish, is known as passive recovery.
> ➤ Recovery through nutrition: Nutrition and hydration are important for recovery.
> ➤ Sleep: One of the most important factors in recovering is getting enough good sleep.

Exercise Nutrition

We'll discuss the significance of replenishing your body's energy stores following exercise, as well as the timing and make-up of post-workout meals and snacks.

Balance of electrolytes and hydration

Electrolyte balance and appropriate hydration are essential for recovery and general health.

slumber and healing

Most of your body's healing and development activities take place during restful sleep. We'll talk about the relationship between fitness and sleep.

Rest Weeks and Rest Days

The significance of including regular rest days and reload weeks in your workout schedule to avoid overtraining and burnout.

Recovery Methods

We'll look at numerous recuperation strategies, such as:

- ➢ Self-myofascial release using foam rolling to alleviate tension in the muscles.
- ➢ Exercises to Increase Flexibility and Decrease Muscle Stiffness Through Stretching and Mobility
- ➢ Reduce inflammation and expedite healing with ice baths and contrast therapy.
- ➢ Professional therapies like massage and bodywork can help you recuperate.

Mental Regrowth

Your mental health is important to your recovery. We'll talk about mental exercises and relaxation techniques to encourage mental renewal.

heeding your body's signals

Learning to pay attention to your body's indications and adapting your workout accordingly is one of the most important components of recovery.

By the end of Chapter 13, you'll realize that recovery is an active phase of your fitness journey rather than a passive one. Using the right recovery strategies can help you complete your tasks, avoid accidents, and achieve long-term success in "Sweat and Success."

Chapter 14

Long-Term Success Strategies for Remaining Committed

In Chapter 14 of "Sweat and Success: A Journey to Fitness," we'll examine the tactics and frame of mind required to uphold your fitness commitment over the long term. Long-term success is accomplished by persevering with your fitness objectives and remaining committed to them.

Long-Term Commitment: Its Power

Long-term commitment to fitness has amazing results, such as better health, more energy, and a higher quality of life. We'll look at why this ongoing dedication is worthwhile.

Having reasonable expectations

Setting attainable goals is essential for long-term success. We'll talk about how to make fitness goals that are both attainable and enduring.

embracing a new way of life

Adopting long-term lifestyle modifications is frequently necessary for long-term success. We'll discuss how to include exercise in your everyday schedule and make it a way of life.

Constructing a Support System

The ability to rely on others can be crucial to maintaining commitment. We'll go over how to build a support system of loved ones, close friends, or those who share your passion for fitness.

Adapting to changes in life

Your fitness path may need to adjust as a result of the many adjustments that life entails. We'll offer tactics for maintaining commitment during significant life changes.

Overcoming Obstacles

Any long-term path inevitably includes setbacks. We'll talk about how to overcome obstacles with tenacity and resolve.

celebrating landmarks

Celebrating your successes on a regular basis, no matter how minor, is essential for maintaining motivation on the arduous path to success.

Having Fun Along the Way

Finding enjoyment in the process is essential for long-term commitment. We'll look at ways to keep your desire and zeal for exercise.

Keeping Current

Maintaining your dedication by keeping up with new trends and research helps keep your exercise education and knowledge current.

Getting Motivated Again

Motivation may fluctuate. We'll talk about ways to get motivated again when you lose it.

seeking advice from a professional

Sometimes consulting a fitness coach, nutritionist, or personal trainer can offer the assistance and direction required for long-term success.

Thinking Back on Your Journey

You can maintain your dedication and recognize your progress by taking some time to think back on your fitness journey.

You'll have a thorough understanding of the tactics and frame of mind required to uphold a long-term commitment to your fitness goals by the end of Chapter 14. You'll continue to thrive in "sweat and success" and lead a better, fitter life for years to come with commitment, adaptability, and a passion for adventure.

Chapter 15

The Next Steps in Continuing Your Fitness Journey

The last chapter of "Sweat and Success: A Journey to Fitness" is Chapter 15, however your lifelong fitness adventure doesn't end here. This chapter will review your accomplishments, provide advice on how to keep them up, and examine the almost limitless opportunities that lie ahead.

Thinking Back on Your Journey

Think back on your progress for a moment. Celebrate your successes and acknowledge the effort and commitment that brought you this far.

Keeping Up Your Progress

Maintaining your fitness goals requires constant effort. We'll talk about how crucial consistency, motivation, and tracking your success are.

Making new objectives

It's time to set new objectives as you accomplish your present ones. We'll look at how to set ambitious yet doable fitness goals to keep your journey interesting.

examining new difficulties

Your physical fitness path can change over time. We'll talk about ways to take on new challenges, including attempting a new sport, competing, or going on a trip.

Adopting a Lifestyle of Fitness

Fitness is a manner of life, not just a destination. We'll offer advice on how to adopt a healthy lifestyle that becomes an essential part of who you are.

Returning favors

Think about ways you might support the fitness industry or encourage others on their adventures. A fulfilling aspect of your fitness journey might be developing into a mentor and role model.

The Fitness of the Future

The fitness industry is always changing. We'll look at new inventions, technology, and trends that could affect your fitness path in the future.

maintaining knowledge and education

It's important to keep learning about fitness and wellness. We'll talk about how to stay current with new findings and advancements.

juggling life and fitness

Your fitness quest shouldn't take priority over other aspects of your life. We'll look at how to juggle your fitness goals with your obligations to your family, job, and other commitments.

Taking Stock of Your Journey

Keep in mind that just getting fit is a wonderful accomplishment. Celebrate both your destination and the amazing journey you took to get there.

Thankfulness and Looking Ahead

Thank fitness for the beneficial changes it has brought about in your life. Keep in mind that your fitness journey is a never-ending, rewarding adventure as you look ahead.

By the time Chapter 15 is through, you'll be eager and optimistic to continue your fitness adventure. You've gone a long way, and the road ahead offers countless chances for development, learning, and self-transformation. Continue your journey in "Sweat and Success," and may your physical fitness endeavors bring you joy, health, and fulfillment for years to come.

Conclusion:

Your Physical Odyssey

I'm happy to hear that you finished "Sweat and Success: A Journey to Fitness." Your journey has been an odyssey full of difficulties, successes, and personal development. Along with changing your physical appearance, you have also developed a stronger, more resilient psyche.

Remember that your fitness journey is a continual and growing story as you stand at this point. Accept the constant chance for development, exploration, and transformation.

Here are a few last ideas to keep in mind as you embark on your fitness odyssey:

➢ You have demonstrated that perseverance is the secret to success. Despite the difficulty of the path, keep moving forward.
➢ Celebrate Your Successes: Consider your successes, no matter how modest they may seem. Honor your progress and the constructive adjustments you've made.

- ➤ Be flexible and receptive to change and development. Adaptability will be your best ally as you set new goals and tackle new challenges.
- ➤ Share your experience, expertise, and enthusiasm with others to inspire them. People close to you can be motivated and inspired by you.
- ➤ Keep learning because the fitness industry is always changing. Keep an open mind and keep learning about new trends, methods, and studies.
- ➤ Recall that enjoying the journey is just as important to health as getting to your final target. Discover happiness, satisfaction, and meaning in each action.
- ➤ Express your gratitude for the health and happiness that working out has given you. Positivity and contentment are fueled by gratitude.

Your fitness odyssey is a lifetime adventure, and there are countless opportunities waiting for you. Continue to write your "Sweat and Success" story while accepting each challenge and celebrating each success. Your journey is a monument to your fortitude, tenacity, and dedication to becoming a fitter, healthier, and more energetic version of yourself. I wish you good health, happiness, and unending success in the years to come.